Mindset Matters

Mindset

MATTERS

Guided journal to help shift your
habits from thought to action

Dr. Charryse Johnson LCMHC NCC

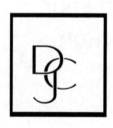

Mindset Matters

Shifting from Thought to Action

ISBN   979-8-9863051-0-3 *Paperback*

Contents

"KNOWLEDGE IS NOT POWER WITHOUT APPLICATION. ARE YOU READY TO ALIGN YOUR EFFORT AND YOUR EXPECATIONS?"
~ DR. CHARRYSE

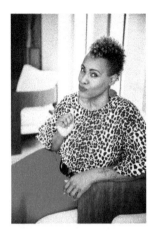

Three essential ingredients for personal growth and change are: clear vision, measurable goals, and building consistent habits. Your habits will either move you towards or away from what you value. Consistent habits also help **rewire the neural pathways** that activate your power of choice.

I've created a 5 on 5 system of success that can shift the trajectory of your life in as little as 25 minutes a day! Small incremental changes allow you to experience success and reduce the potential for overwhelm.

Greatness lives inside of you!

7 Signs You're Standing In Your Own Way

- You're not a priority in your own life.

- You spend more time focused on other people's business than your own.

- You constantly compare your progress to others.

- You struggle with consistency and lack genuine dedication to your goals.

- You manage yourself like a liability instead of an asset

- You let your external world dictate your internal state of being.

- You have an excuse for everything.

Turn the page and commit to practicing mindful intention, one moment, one day at a time. There's no need to look back or recall moments where you've failed in the past.

The path forward requires your full participation. Let the knowledge of your past become the inspiration for your future! *I believe in you!*

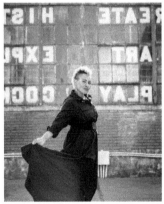

Better is possible!

5
ON 5 SYSTEM OF SUCCESS

The foundation of the 5 on 5 system is to work through all 5 components, for 5 minutes a day, 5 or many days a week. Keeping each practice to 5 minutes *eliminates excuses around not having enough time.* Remember, the way forward is to create a life you don't want to escape.

#1: REVIEW YOUR DAY

Before you start saving the world, stop and review your schedule for the day. Consider how it matches up with the current context of your life. For example, if you have young children or you're a caretaker, changes may be needed to compensate for your energy level. This practice helps you cultivate the *power to run your day* instead of allowing your day to run you. Soon, you'll recognize the benefit of prioritizing and honoring your needs first.

#2: PERSONAL DEVELOPMENT

Use this time to implement a positive message that helps you shift how you think and move forward with new insight. This time is intended to support personal goals you've set for yourself. This could include listening to a podcast, reading a book, or watching part of a video that supports the vision you have for yourself.

#3: SESSION OF SILENCE

The ultimate goal is to spend five minutes engaged in deep breathing, stillness, and silence — *during the day*. If complete silence is daunting, start with playing instrumental music in the background. I highly recommend bilateral or binaural music through headphones. This practice helps you check in, self-regulate and recalibrate your emotions. It's time to resist the rhythm of the rush and make adjustments that will help reduce your stress. Unchecked stress activates your nervous system, is viewed as danger by the brain, and can encourage decisions based on impulse and survival. Nourish your nervous system!

#4: GRATITUDE

Research demonstrates when we operate from a place of gratitude and we choose to bring up the things we are thankful to experience, it changes the chemistry of our brain and instills a sense of hope. Even if you write the same things for a few weeks, that's ok! This is a powerful practice to help you unlearn discounting the positive and focus on what needs to be better. Every time you *choose* to exercise gratitude, you reduce the brain's natural negativity bias. You could even practice this as a family!

#5 EVALUATE YOUR DAY

At the end of the day, identify *what you did well* and what you're looking forward to experiencing in the days to come. If you notice there's nothing to look forward to, you may benefit from creating a new reality. The second component of this practice is checking in with an accountability partner and being honest about the progress you're making (or not making) towards your goals. This is an opportunity to unmask and to make sure you're using every resource and tool that supports your goals.

To round out your day, I've created a few components to increase your mind-body integration. There's space to **track your sleep, track your water intake, and practice mindful eating.**

Mindful eating is the practice of fully engaging in your eating experience, and honoring your hunger and fullness. You'll also have a chance to identify if you're eating to **NOURISH or NUMB.**

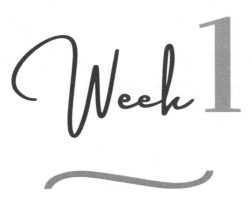

Doctor's Note

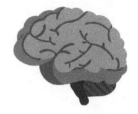

Slowing down is an essential part of taking action and honoring your choices. Adjust your pace, but don't stop running your race. There will undoubtedly be moments that try to knock you off your rhythm, but find the new beat and keep moving.

**MAKE
ADJUSTMENTS
AS NEEDED**

-Dr. Charryse

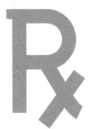

Prescription for: Growth

#protectyourpeace

Date: Week 1

Patient: _____

Instructions:

At least once this week, set and communicate a boundary that supports your goals. Try to keep your words simple, concise, and unapologetic. You may feel anxious or guilty, but with practice those reactions will lighten.

Refill script_____times

x - PRN NR

Sleep

I woke up feeling...   **Hrs:**

_____

_____   1 2 3 4 5 6 7 8+

_____

_____

Review your day: **Water**

**What adjustments
to your schedule
would honor your
needs today?**   16 16 16 16

16 16 16 16

_____

_____   Personal
development:
_____

_____   _____

**What do you want to
experience today?**   _____

_____   _____

_____   _____

_____   _____

_____   _____

_____

Gratitude:

_____

_____

_____

5 min of meditation, stillness, or quiet

1   2   3   4   5

Be mindful of your eating

_____

_____

_____

_____

Evaluate your day. What went well today?

_____

_____

_____

_____

Today my eating motivation was to...

NOURISH

NUMB

Tomorrow I look forward to...

_____

_____

_____

_____

☐   _used an accountability resource_

Daily Reflections

Scripture of the day:

Isaiah 41:10

Sleep

I woke up feeling...   **Hrs:**

_____
_____   1 2 3 4 5 6 7 8+
_____
_____
_____

Review your day: **Water**

**What adjustments
to your schedule
would honor your
needs today?**

16 16 16 16

16 16 16 16

_____
_____
_____
_____

**Personal
development:**

**What do you want to
experience today?**

_____
_____
_____
_____
_____
_____
_____
_____

Gratitude:

_____

_____

_____

_____

5 min of meditation,
stillness, or quiet

1 2   3 4 5

_Be mindful of
your eating_

_____

_____

_____

_____

**Evaluate your day.
What went well
today?**

_____

_____

_____

_____

**Today my eating
motivation was to...**

NOURISH

NUMB

Tomorrow I look
forward to...

_____

_____

_____

_____

☐   _used an accountability resource_

Daily Reflections

_____

_____

_____

_____

_____

_____

_____

_____

_____

_____

Scripture of the day:

John 16:33

Sleep

I woke up feeling...

Hrs:

_____
_____   1 2 3 4 5 6 7 8+
_____
_____
_____

Review your day:

Water

What adjustments to your schedule would honor your needs today?

16 16 16 16

16 16 16 16

_____
_____
_____
_____

Personal
development:

_____

What do you want to experience today?

_____
_____

_____

_____
_____
_____

_____

_____

Gratitude:

_____

_____

_____

_____

5 min of meditation, stillness, or quiet

1 2   3 4 5

Be mindful of your eating

_____

_____

_____

_____

Evaluate your day. What went well today?

_____

_____

_____

_____

Today my eating motivation was to...

NOURISH

NUMB

Tomorrow I look forward to...

_____

_____

_____

_____

☐   *used an accountability resource*

Daily Reflections

_____

_____

_____

_____

_____

_____

_____

_____

_____

_____

_____

Scripture of the day:

Psalm 46:11

Sleep

I woke up feeling...

Hrs:

_____
_____
_____
_____
_____

1 2 3 4 5

Review your day:

Water

What adjustments to your schedule would honor your needs today?

16 16 16 16

16 16 16 16

_____
_____
_____
_____

Personal development:

What do you want to experience today?

_____
_____
_____
_____
_____
_____
_____
_____
_____

Gratitude:

_____

_____

_____

_____

5 min of meditation, stillness, or quiet

1 2   3 4 5

Be mindful of your eating

_____

_____

_____

_____

Evaluate your day. What went well today?

_____

_____

_____

_____

Today my eating motivation was to...

NOURISH

NUMB

Tomorrow I look forward to...

_____

_____

_____

_____

☐   _used an accountability resource_

Daily Reflections

_____

_____

_____

_____

_____

_____

_____

_____

_____

_____

Scripture of the day:

Thessalonians 3:13

Sleep

I woke up feeling...

Hrs:

_____

_____

1 2 3 4 5 6 7 8+

_____

_____

Review your day:

Water

What adjustments to your schedule would honor your needs today?

16 16 16 16

16 16 16 16

_____

_____

_____

Personal development:

_____

_____

What do you want to experience today?

_____

_____

_____

_____

_____

_____

_____

_____

Gratitude:

_____

_____

_____

5 min of meditation, stillness, or quiet

1 2   3   4   5

Be mindful of your eating

_____

_____

_____

Evaluate your day. What went well today?

_____

_____

_____

Today my eating motivation was to...

NOURISH

NUMB

Tomorrow I look forward to...

_____

_____

_____

_____

☐   _used an accountability resource_

Daily Reflections

_____

_____

_____

_____

_____

_____

_____

_____

_____

_____

Scripture of the day:

2 Chronicles 32:7

Sleep

I woke up feeling...   **Hrs:**

_____
_____   1 2 3 4 5 6 7 8+
_____
_____

Review your day: **Water**

What adjustments   16 16 16 16
to your schedule
would honor your
needs today?   16 16 16 16

_____
_____
_____   Personal
_____   development:

                                 _____
What do you want to   _____
experience today?   _____

_____   _____
_____   _____
_____   _____
_____   _____

Gratitude:

_____

_____

_____

_____

5 min of meditation,
stillness, or quiet

1 2   3 4 5

_Be mindful of
your eating_

_____

_____

_____

_____

**Evaluate your day.
What went well
today?**

_____

_____

_____

_____

**Today my eating
motivation was to...**

NOURISH

NUMB

Tomorrow I look
forward to...

_____

_____

_____

_____

☐   _used an accountability resource_

Daily Reflections

_____

_____

_____

_____

_____

_____

_____

_____

_____

_____

_____

Scripture of the day:

Philippians 4:13

Sleep

I woke up feeling...

Hrs:

_____

_____

1 2 3 4 5 6 7 8+

_____

_____

Review your day:

Water

What adjustments to your schedule would honor your needs today?

16 16 16 16

16 16 16 16

_____

_____

_____

Personal development:

_____

_____

What do you want to experience today?

_____

_____

_____

_____

_____

_____

_____

_____

_____

Gratitude:

5 min of meditation,
stillness, or quiet

1 2   3 4 5

Be mindful of
your eating

Evaluate your day.
What went well
today?

Today my eating
motivation was to...

Tomorrow I look
forward to...

NOURISH

NUMB

☐   _used an accountability resource_

Daily Reflections

_____

_____

_____

_____

_____

_____

_____

_____

_____

_____

Scripture of the day:

1 Chronicles 22:13

Week 2

Doctor's *Note*

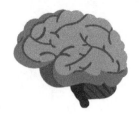

Sometimes our body can be conditioned to respond in ways that are no longer true. As you continue to engage in these daily practices, you will have greater awareness of your autonomic habits. If you find yourself in the middle of some old patterns, *acknowledge it and pivot*. You've made it through everything that's come your way, and I fully believe you'll conquer what lies ahead.

YOU ARE BREAKING THE CYCLE!

—Dr. Charryse

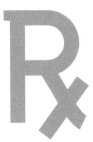

Prescription for: Growth

#bepresent

Date: Week 2

Patient: _____

Instructions: _____

Power off your phone and go on a *mindful walk*. As you walk, focus on matching each breath to each step. Then, slowly tune in to the sights and sounds around you. Notice how it feels to be present in nature.

Refill script_____times

x – PRN NR

Sleep   Date: _____

I woke up feeling...   **Hrs:**

_____
                          1 2 3 4 5 6 7 8+
_____

_____

_____

Review your day: **Water**

**What adjustments
to your schedule**   16 16 16 16
**would honor your
needs today?**   16 16 16 16

_____
_____
_____
                                    **Personal
_____   development:**

What do you want to   _____
experience today?   _____

_____   _____

_____   _____

_____   _____

_____   _____

Gratitude:

_____

_____

_____

_____

5 min of meditation,
stillness, or quiet

1   2   3   4   5

*Be mindful of
your eating*

_____

_____

_____

_____

**Evaluate your day.
What went well
today?**

_____

_____

_____

_____

**Today my eating
motivation was to...**

NOURISH

NUMB

Tomorrow I look
forward to...

_____

_____

_____

_____

☐   *used an accountability resource*

Daily Reflections

_____

_____

_____

_____

_____

_____

_____

_____

_____

_____

Scripture of the day:

Philippians 1:28

Sleep

I woke up feeling...   **Hrs:**

_____

_____   1 2 3 4 5 6 7 8+

_____

_____

Review your day: **Water**

What adjustments
to your schedule   16 16 16 16
would honor your
needs today?   16 16 16 16

_____

_____

_____
                                        Personal
_____   development:

                              _____

What do you want to   _____
experience today?
                              _____

_____

_____   _____

_____   _____

_____

_____   _____

Gratitude:

_____

_____

_____

5 min of meditation,
stillness, or quiet

1 2   3   4   5

*Be mindful of
your eating*

_____

_____

_____

_____

**Evaluate your day.
What went well
today?**

_____

_____

_____

_____

**Today my eating
motivation was to...**

NOURISH

NUMB

Tomorrow I look
forward to...

_____

_____

_____

_____

☐   *used an accountability resource*

Daily Reflections

_____

_____

_____

_____

_____

_____

_____

_____

_____

_____

_____

Scripture of the day:

Ephesians 6:10-18

Sleep

I woke up feeling...

Hrs:

_____
_____
_____
_____

1 2 3 4 5 6 7 8+

Review your day:

Water

What adjustments to your schedule would honor your needs today?

16 16 16 16

16 16 16 16

_____
_____
_____
_____

Personal development:

What do you want to experience today?

_____
_____
_____
_____

_____
_____
_____
_____

Gratitude:

_____

_____

_____

5 min of meditation,
stillness, or quiet

1 2 3 4 5

*Be mindful of
your eating*

_____

_____

_____

_____

**Evaluate your day.
What went well
today?**

_____

_____

_____

_____

**Today my eating
motivation was to...**

NOURISH

NUMB

Tomorrow I look
forward to...

_____

_____

_____

_____

☐   *used an accountability resource*

Daily Reflections

_____

_____

_____

_____

_____

_____

_____

_____

_____

_____

Scripture of the day:

Zephaniah 3:17

Sleep

I woke up feeling...

Hrs:

1 2 3 4 5 6 7 8+

_____

_____

_____

_____

_____

Review your day:

What adjustments to your schedule would honor your needs today?

Water

16 16 16 16

16 16 16 16

_____

_____

_____

_____

Personal development:

_____

What do you want to experience today?

_____

_____

_____

_____

_____

_____

_____

_____

Gratitude:

_____

_____

_____

_____

5 min of meditation,
stillness, or quiet

1 2   3 4 5

*Be mindful of
your eating*

_____

_____

_____

_____

**Evaluate your day.
What went well
today?**

_____

_____

_____

_____

**Today my eating
motivation was to...**

NOURISH

NUMB

Tomorrow I look
forward to...

_____

_____

_____

_____

☐   *used an accountability resource*

Daily Reflections

_____

_____

_____

_____

_____

_____

_____

_____

_____

_____

_____

Scripture of the day:

Romans 15:13

Sleep

I woke up feeling...

Hrs:

_____

_____

1 2 3 4 5 6 7 8+

_____

_____

_____

Review your day:

Water

What adjustments to your schedule would honor your needs today?

16 16 16 16

16 16 16 16

_____

_____

_____

_____

Personal
development:

_____

What do you want to experience today?

_____

_____

_____

_____

_____

_____

_____

_____

Gratitude:

_____

_____

_____

5 min of meditation, stillness, or quiet

1 2   3 4 5

Be mindful of your eating

_____

_____

_____

_____

Evaluate your day. What went well today?

_____

_____

_____

_____

Today my eating motivation was to...

NOURISH

NUMB

Tomorrow I look forward to...

_____

_____

_____

_____

☐   _used an accountability resource_

Daily Reflections

_____

_____

_____

_____

_____

_____

_____

_____

_____

_____

Scripture of the day:

1 John 4:18

Sleep

I woke up feeling...   **Hrs:**

_____

_____   1 2 3 4 5 6 7 8+

_____

_____

_____

Review your day: **Water**

**What adjustments
to your schedule
would honor your
needs today?**   16 16 16 16

16 16 16 16

_____

_____

_____   Personal

_____   development:

_____

**What do you want to
experience today?**   _____

_____

_____   _____

_____

_____   _____

_____

_____   _____

Gratitude:

_____

_____

_____

_____

5 min of meditation, stillness, or quiet

1 2 3 4 5

Be mindful of your eating

_____

_____

_____

_____

Evaluate your day. What went well today?

_____

_____

_____

_____

Today my eating motivation was to...

NOURISH

NUMB

Tomorrow I look forward to...

_____

_____

_____

_____

☐   *used an accountability resource*

Daily Reflections

_____

_____

_____

_____

_____

_____

_____

_____

_____

_____

Scripture of the day:

2 Chronicles 32:8

Sleep

I woke up feeling...   **Hrs:**

_____

_____   1 2 3 4 5 6 7 8+

_____

_____

Review your day: **Water**

**What adjustments
to your schedule
would honor your
needs today?**   16 16 16 16

                      16 16 16 16

_____

_____

_____   Personal
                                        development:

_____
                              _____
**What do you want to
experience today?**   _____

_____   _____

_____   _____

_____   _____

_____   _____

_____

Gratitude:

_____
_____
_____
_____

5 min of meditation,
stillness, or quiet

1 2   3 4 5

_Be mindful of
your eating_

_____
_____
_____
_____

**Evaluate your day.
What went well
today?**

_____
_____
_____
_____

**Today my eating
motivation was to...**

NOURISH

NUMB

Tomorrow I look
forward to...

_____
_____
_____
_____

☐   _used an accountability resource_

Daily Reflections

_____

_____

_____

_____

_____

_____

_____

_____

_____

_____

Scripture of the day:

Matthew 11:28

Week 3

Doctor's Note

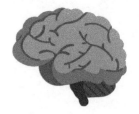

Every time we push through our pain without addressing the root, we lock those experiences into our procedural memory. These memories can silently control how we think and respond. It's important to *heal* what lies beneath the surface.

YOU BECOME WHAT YOU BELIEVE!

-Dr. Charryse

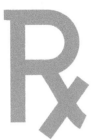

Prescription for: Growth

#selftalk

Date: Week 3

Patient: _____

Instructions:

Give yourself daily compliments. Write them down or say them out loud while you look in the mirror. Center these compliments around *who you are*, not what you do.

Refill script_____times

x – PRN NR

Sleep

I woke up feeling...   **Hrs:**

_____

_____   1 2 3 4 5 6 7 8+

_____

_____

Review your day: **Water**

**What adjustments
to your schedule
would honor your
needs today?**

16 16 16 16

16 16 16 16

_____

_____

_____   **Personal
development:**

_____

**What do you want to
experience today?**

_____

_____

_____

_____

_____

_____

_____

_____

Gratitude:

_____

_____

_____

5 min of meditation,
stillness, or quiet

1 2   3   4   5

*Be mindful of
your eating*

**Evaluate your day.
What went well
today?**

**Today my eating
motivation was to...**

NOURISH

NUMB

Tomorrow I look
forward to...

☐   *used an accountability resource*

Daily Reflections

_____

_____

_____

_____

_____

_____

_____

_____

_____

_____

Scripture of the day:

1 Corinthians 15:58

Sleep

I woke up feeling...   **Hrs:**

_____

_____   1 2 3 4 5 6 7 8+

_____

_____

Review your day: **Water**

What adjustments
to your schedule   16 16 16 16
would honor your
needs today?   16 16 16 16

_____

_____

_____   Personal
                              development:
_____

                              _____

What do you want to   _____
experience today?
                              _____
_____
                              _____
_____
                              _____
_____
                              _____
_____
                              _____
_____

Gratitude:

_____

_____

_____

_____

5 min of meditation, stillness, or quiet

1 2   3 4 5

Be mindful of your eating

_____

_____

_____

_____

Evaluate your day. What went well today?

_____

_____

_____

_____

Today my eating motivation was to...

NOURISH

NUMB

Tomorrow I look forward to...

_____

_____

_____

_____

☐   _used an accountability resource_

Daily Reflections

_____

_____

_____

_____

_____

_____

_____

_____

_____

_____

Scripture of the day:

Luke 12:4

Sleep

I woke up feeling...   **Hrs:**

_____

_____   1 2 3 4 5 6 7 8+

_____

_____

Review your day: **Water**

**What adjustments
to your schedule   16 16 16 16
would honor your
needs today?**   16 16 16 16

_____

_____

_____

_____   Personal
                                     development:

                                     _____

**What do you want to   _____
experience today?**

                                     _____

_____

_____   _____

_____

_____   _____

_____

Gratitude:

_____

_____

_____

5 min of meditation,
stillness, or quiet

1 2   3   4   5

_Be mindful of
your eating_

Evaluate your day.
**What went well
today?**

**Today my eating
motivation was to...**

Tomorrow I look
forward to...

NOURISH

NUMB

☐ _used an accountability resource_

Daily Reflections

_____

_____

_____

_____

_____

_____

_____

_____

_____

_____

_____

_____

_____

_____

_____

Scripture of the day:

Psalm 118:14-16

Sleep

I woke up feeling...

Hrs:

1 2 3 4 5 6 7 8+

_____
_____
_____
_____
_____

Review your day:

Water

What adjustments
to your schedule
would honor your
needs today?

16 16 16 16

16 16 16 16

_____
_____
_____
_____

Personal
development:

_____

**What do you want to
experience today?**

_____
_____
_____
_____
_____
_____
_____
_____

Gratitude:

_____

_____

_____

_____

5 min of meditation, stillness, or quiet

1 2   3 4 5

Be mindful of your eating

_____

_____

_____

_____

Evaluate your day. What went well today?

_____

_____

_____

_____

Today my eating motivation was to...

NOURISH

NUMB

Tomorrow I look forward to...

_____

_____

_____

_____

☐   *used an accountability resource*

Daily Reflections

_____

_____

_____

_____

_____

_____

_____

_____

_____

_____

_____

Scripture of the day:

John 14:27

Sleep

I woke up feeling...   **Hrs:**

_____

_____   1 2 3 4 5 6 7 8+

_____

_____

Review your day: **Water**

**What adjustments
to your schedule
would honor your
needs today?**

16 16 16 16

16 16 16 16

_____

_____

_____   **Personal
development:**

_____

**What do you want to
experience today?**

_____

_____

_____

_____

_____

_____

_____

_____

Gratitude:

_____

_____

_____

_____

5 min of meditation,
stillness, or quiet

1 2   3   4   5

Be mindful of
your eating

_____

_____

_____

_____

Evaluate your day.
What went well
today?

_____

_____

_____

_____

Today my eating
motivation was to...

NOURISH

NUMB

Tomorrow I look
forward to...

_____

_____

_____

_____

☐   *used an accountability resource*

Daily Reflections

_____

_____

_____

_____

_____

_____

_____

_____

_____

_____

_____

Scripture of the day:

Deuteronomy 31:6

Sleep

I woke up feeling...　　　　　　　**Hrs:**

_____

_____　　1 2 3 4 5 6 7 8+

_____

_____

Review your day:　　　　　　**Water**

**What adjustments
to your schedule
would honor your
needs today?**　　　　16 16 16 16

　　　　　　　　　　16 16 16 16

_____

_____

_____

_____

　　　　　　　　　　　*Personal
development:*

_____

**What do you want to
experience today?**

_____

_____

_____

_____

_____

_____

Gratitude:

_____

_____

_____

5 min of meditation, stillness, or quiet

1 2   3 4 5

Be mindful of your eating

Evaluate your day. What went well today?

Today my eating motivation was to...

NOURISH

NUMB

Tomorrow I look forward to...

☐   _used an accountability resource_

Daily Reflections

_____

_____

_____

_____

_____

_____

_____

_____

_____

_____

Scripture of the day:

1 Corinthians 16:13

Sleep

I woke up feeling...

Hrs:

1 2 3 4 5 6 7 8+

_____

_____

_____

_____

Review your day:

**What adjustments
to your schedule
would honor your
needs today?**

Water

16 16 16 16

16 16 16 16

_____

_____

_____

Personal
development:

_____

_____

**What do you want to
experience today?**

_____

_____

_____

_____

_____

_____

_____

_____

Gratitude:

_____

_____

_____

5 min of meditation,
stillness, or quiet

1 2   3 4 5

*Be mindful of
your eating*

_____

_____

_____

_____

**Evaluate your day.
What went well
today?**

_____

_____

_____

_____

**Today my eating
motivation was to...**

NOURISH

NUMB

Tomorrow I look
forward to...

_____

_____

_____

_____

☐   *used an accountability resource*

Daily Reflections

_____

_____

_____

_____

_____

_____

_____

_____

_____

_____

Scripture of the day:

Proverbs 3:5-6

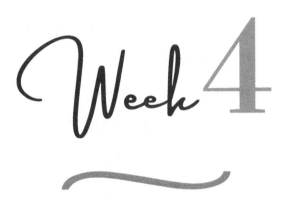

Week 4

Doctor's *Note*

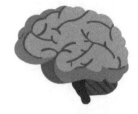

How we respond to our position is dictated by our perspective. When life is viewed through the lens of doubt, we become paralyzed. We stop taking action and no longer believe our effort has value. Wake up, dear one! Reposition your eyes, focus on your *why* and stop hitting snooze! Your purpose doesn't change when storms come your way.

FOCUS FORWARD AND MAINTAIN HOPE!

-Dr. Charryse

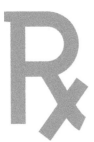 **Prescription for: Growth**

#treatyoself

Date: <u>Week 4</u>

Patient: _____

Instructions:

Rewards boost dopamine, a neurotransmitter that makes your brain happy. This week identify an item, activity, or experience that would bring you joy. Make it *happen*, regardless of any guilt you may feel.

Refill script_____times

x – PRN NR

Sleep

I woke up feeling...   **Hrs:**

_____

_____   1 2 3 4 5 6 7 8+

_____

_____

_____

Review your day: **Water**

**What adjustments
to your schedule
would honor your
needs today?**   16 16 16 16

                        16 16 16 16

_____

_____

_____   **Personal
development:**

_____

**What do you want to
experience today?**   _____

                        _____

_____   _____

_____   _____

_____   _____

_____   _____

Gratitude:

_____

_____

_____

_____

5 min of meditation, stillness, or quiet

1 2   3   4   5

Be mindful of your eating

_____

_____

_____

_____

Evaluate your day. What went well today?

_____

_____

_____

_____

Today my eating motivation was to...

NOURISH

NUMB

Tomorrow I look forward to...

_____

_____

_____

_____

☐   _used an accountability resource_

Daily Reflections

_____

_____

_____

_____

_____

_____

_____

_____

_____

_____

_____

Scripture of the day:

1 Corinthians 10:13

Sleep

I woke up feeling...   **Hrs:**

_____

_____   1 2 3 4 5 6 7 8+

_____

_____

Review your day: **Water**

**What adjustments
to your schedule
would honor your
needs today?**   16 16 16 16

16 16 16 16

_____

_____

_____   Personal
development:
_____

_____

**What do you want to
experience today?**   _____

_____   _____

_____   _____

_____   _____

_____   _____

Gratitude:

_____
_____
_____

5 min of meditation, stillness, or quiet

1 2   3 4 5

Be mindful of your eating

Evaluate your day. What went well today?

_____
_____
_____

_____
_____
_____

Today my eating motivation was to...

NOURISH

NUMB

Tomorrow I look forward to...

_____
_____
_____

☐   _used an accountability resource_

Daily Reflections

_____

_____

_____

_____

_____

_____

_____

_____

_____

_____

Scripture of the day:

Isaiah 12:2

Sleep

I woke up feeling...

Hrs:

_____

_____

1 2 3 4 5 6 7 8+

_____

_____

Review your day:

Water

**What adjustments
to your schedule
would honor your
needs today?**

16 16 16 16

16 16 16 16

_____

_____

_____

_____

**Personal
development:**

**What do you want to
experience today?**

_____

_____

_____

_____

_____

_____

_____

_____

Gratitude:

_____

_____

_____

5 min of meditation,
stillness, or quiet

1 2   3   4   5

*Be mindful of
your eating*

_____

_____

_____

**Evaluate your day.
What went well
today?**

_____

_____

_____

**Today my eating
motivation was to...**

NOURISH

NUMB

Tomorrow I look
forward to...

_____

_____

_____

☐   *used an accountability resource*

Daily Reflections

Scripture of the day:

Psalm 16:8

Sleep   Date: _____

I woke up feeling...   **Hrs:**

_____
_____   1 2 3 4 5 6 7 8+
_____
_____

Review your day: **Water**

**What adjustments
to your schedule**   16 16 16 16
**would honor your
needs today?**   16 16 16 16

_____
_____
_____   Personal
_____   development:

                                             _____
What do you want to   _____
experience today?   _____

_____   _____
_____   _____
_____   _____
_____   _____

Gratitude:

_____

_____

_____

_____

Be mindful of your eating

_____

_____

_____

_____

Evaluate your day. What went well today?

_____

_____

_____

_____

Today my eating motivation was to...

NOURISH

NUMB

Tomorrow I look forward to...

_____

_____

_____

_____

☐   *used an accountability resource*

Daily Reflections

_____

_____

_____

_____

_____

_____

_____

_____

_____

_____

Scripture of the day:

2 Corinthians 4:16-18

Sleep

I woke up feeling...   **Hrs:**

_____

_____   1 2 3 4 5 6 7 8+

_____

_____

_____

Review your day: **Water**

**What adjustments
to your schedule
would honor your
needs today?**   16 16 16 16

                                            16 16 16 16

_____

_____

_____   **Personal
                                  development:**

_____   _____

**What do you want to
experience today?**   _____

_____   _____

_____   _____

_____   _____

_____   _____

_____

Gratitude:

_____

_____

_____

_____

5 min of meditation,
stillness, or quiet

1 2   3   4   5

_Be mindful of
your eating_

_____

_____

_____

_____

**Evaluate your day.
What went well
today?**

_____

_____

_____

_____

**Today my eating
motivation was to...**

NOURISH

NUMB

Tomorrow I look
forward to...

_____

_____

_____

_____

☐   _used an accountability resource_

Daily Reflections

Scripture of the day:

Ezra 10:4

Sleep

I woke up feeling...

Hrs:

_____

_____   1 2 3 4 5 6 7 8+

_____

_____

Review your day: **Water**

**What adjustments
to your schedule
would honor your
needs today?**

16 16 16 16

16 16 16 16

_____

_____

_____   **Personal
development:**

**What do you want to
experience today?**

_____

_____

_____

_____

_____

_____

_____

_____

Gratitude:

_____

_____

_____

_____

5 min of meditation, stillness, or quiet

1 2 3 4 5

Be mindful of your eating

_____

_____

_____

_____

Evaluate your day. What went well today?

_____

_____

_____

_____

Today my eating motivation was to...

NOURISH

NUMB

Tomorrow I look forward to...

_____

_____

_____

_____

☐   _used an accountability resource_

Daily Reflections

_____

_____

_____

_____

_____

_____

_____

_____

_____

_____

_____

Scripture of the day:

Philippians 1:27

Sleep

I woke up feeling... **Hrs:**

_____

_____ 1 2 3 4 5 6 7 8+

_____

_____

Review your day: **Water**

**What adjustments
to your schedule
would honor your
needs today?**

16 16 16 16

16 16 16 16

_____

_____

_____ **Personal
development:**

_____

_____

**What do you want to
experience today?** _____

_____

_____

_____

_____

_____

_____

Gratitude:

_____

_____

_____

5 min of meditation,
stillness, or quiet

1 2   3 4 5

Be mindful of
your eating

_____

_____

_____

_____

Evaluate your day.
What went well
today?

_____

_____

_____

_____

Today my eating
motivation was to...

NOURISH

NUMB

Tomorrow I look
forward to...

_____

_____

_____

_____

☐   *used an accountability resource*

Daily Reflections

Scripture of the day:

Psalm 18:1-2

Week 5

Doctor's Note

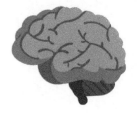

No matter how many goals you set, leave perfection off the list. It's an illusion, a never ending pursuit that robs you of gratitude. Walk boldly into the weeks ahead knowing that every day is a new opportunity to develop your identity.

PROGRESS OVER PERFECTION!

-Dr. Charryse

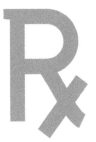 **Prescription for: Growth**

#embodyhealing

Date: Week 5

Patient: _____

Instructions:

Engage in mindful exercise by focusing on the sensations in your body while it moves. For example, mentally scanning your body and thinking about the muscle groups that are engaged can bring peace to a wandering mind. Practice this 2-3x this week for at least ten minutes.

Refill Script_____times

x – PRN NR

Sleep

I woke up feeling...

Hrs:

_____

_____

_____

_____

1 2 3 4 5 6 7 8+

Review your day:

Water

What adjustments to your schedule would honor your needs today?

16 16 16 16

16 16 16 16

_____

_____

_____

_____

Personal development:

_____

What do you want to experience today?

_____

_____

_____

_____

_____

_____

_____

_____

_____

Gratitude:

_____

_____

_____

5 min of meditation,
stillness, or quiet

1 2   3   4   5

*Be mindful of
your eating*

_____

_____

_____

_____

**Evaluate your day.
What went well
today?**

_____

_____

_____

_____

**Today my eating
motivation was to...**

NOURISH

NUMB

Tomorrow I look
forward to...

_____

_____

_____

_____

☐   *used an accountability resource*

Daily Reflections

_____

_____

_____

_____

_____

_____

_____

_____

_____

_____

_____

Scripture of the day:

2 Samuel 10:12

Sleep

I woke up feeling...   **Hrs:**

_____
_____   1 2 3 4 5 6 7 8+
_____
_____

Review your day: **Water**

What adjustments
to your schedule   16 16 16 16
would honor your
needs today?   16 16 16 16

_____
_____
_____
_____   Personal
                              development:

                              _____
What do you want to   _____
experience today?   _____
_____   _____
_____   _____
_____   _____
_____   _____
_____

Gratitude:

_____

_____

_____

5 min of meditation,
stillness, or quiet

1   2   3   4   5

_Be mindful of
your eating_

**Evaluate your day.
What went well
today?**

**Today my eating
motivation was to...**

NOURISH

NUMB

Tomorrow I look
forward to...

☐   _used an accountability resource_

Daily Reflections

_____

_____

_____

_____

_____

_____

_____

_____

_____

_____

_____

_____

Scripture of the day:

Galatians 6:9

Sleep

I woke up feeling...   **Hrs:**

_____

_____   1 2 3 4 5 6 7 8+

_____

_____

_____

Review your day: **Water**

**What adjustments
to your schedule**   16 16 16 16
**would honor your
needs today?**   16 16 16 16

_____

_____

_____

_____
                                                    Personal
                                                development:

What do you want to   _____
experience today?
                                      _____

_____   _____

_____   _____

_____   _____

_____   _____

Gratitude:

_____

_____

_____

5 min of meditation,
stillness, or quiet

1 2   3   4   5

*Be mindful of
your eating*

_____

_____

_____

**Evaluate your day.
What went well
today?**

_____

_____

_____

**Today my eating
motivation was to...**

NOURISH

NUMB

Tomorrow I look
forward to...

_____

_____

_____

☐   *used an accountability resource*

Daily Reflections

_____

_____

_____

_____

_____

_____

_____

_____

_____

_____

Scripture of the day:

Jeremiah 29:11

Sleep

I woke up feeling...

Hrs:

_____
_____

1 2 3 4 5 6 7 8+

_____
_____

Review your day:

Water

**What adjustments
to your schedule
would honor your
needs today?**

16 16 16 16

16 16 16 16

_____
_____
_____
_____

Personal
development:

_____

**What do you want to
experience today?**

_____
_____
_____
_____

_____
_____
_____
_____

Gratitude:

_____

_____

_____

5 min of meditation,
stillness, or quiet

1 2 3 4 5

*Be mindful of
your eating*

**Evaluate your day.
What went well
today?**

_____

_____

_____

**Today my eating
motivation was to...**

NOURISH

NUMB

Tomorrow I look
forward to...

_____

_____

_____

☐ *used an accountability resource*

Daily Reflections

_____

_____

_____

_____

_____

_____

_____

_____

_____

_____

Scripture of the day:

Isaiah 26:3

Sleep

I woke up feeling...

Hrs:

_____

_____

1 2 3 4 5 6 7 8+

_____

_____

_____

Review your day:

Water

**What adjustments
to your schedule
would honor your
needs today?**

16 16 16 16

16 16 16 16

_____

_____

_____

_____

Personal
development:

_____

**What do you want to
experience today?**

_____

_____

_____

_____

_____

_____

_____

_____

Gratitude:

_____

_____

_____

5 min of meditation,
stillness, or quiet

1 2   3 4 5

*Be mindful of
your eating*

_____

_____

_____

**Evaluate your day.
What went well
today?**

_____

_____

_____

**Today my eating
motivation was to...**

NOURISH

NUMB

Tomorrow I look
forward to...

_____

_____

_____

_____

☐   *used an accountability resource*

Daily Reflections

_____

_____

_____

_____

_____

_____

_____

_____

_____

_____

Scripture of the day:

2 Timothy 1:7

Sleep

I woke up feeling...

Hrs:

_____

_____

1 2 3 4 5 6 7 8+

_____

_____

_____

Review your day:

Water

What adjustments to your schedule would honor your needs today?

16 16 16 16

16 16 16 16

_____

_____

_____

Personal development:

_____

What do you want to experience today?

_____

_____

_____

_____

_____

_____

_____

_____

Gratitude:

_____
_____
_____
_____

5 min of meditation, stillness, or quiet

1 2   3 4 5

Be mindful of your eating

_____
_____
_____
_____

Evaluate your day. What went well today?

_____
_____
_____
_____

Today my eating motivation was to...

NOURISH

NUMB

Tomorrow I look forward to...

_____
_____
_____
_____

☐   _used an accountability resource_

Daily Reflections

_____

_____

_____

_____

_____

_____

_____

_____

_____

_____

Scripture of the day:

Colossians 3:15

Sleep

I woke up feeling...

Hrs:

1 2 3 4 5 6 7 8+

_____
_____
_____
_____
_____

Review your day:

Water

What adjustments to your schedule would honor your needs today?

16 16 16 16

16 16 16 16

_____
_____
_____
_____

Personal development:

_____
_____
_____

What do you want to experience today?

_____
_____
_____
_____
_____
_____
_____

Gratitude:

_____

_____

_____

5 min of meditation,
stillness, or quiet

1 2   3   4   5

Be mindful of
your eating

_____

_____

_____

_____

Evaluate your day.
What went well
today?

_____

_____

_____

_____

Today my eating
motivation was to...

NOURISH

NUMB

Tomorrow I look
forward to...

_____

_____

_____

_____

☐   *used an accountability resource*

Daily Reflections

_____

_____

_____

_____

_____

_____

_____

_____

_____

_____

Scripture of the day:

Psalm 27:1

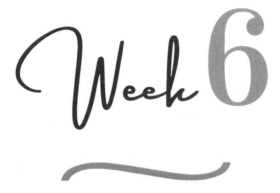

Week 6

Doctor's Note

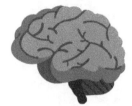

Making peace with your body doesn't mean abandoning your vision for health. It means treating yourself with compassion and being mindful that your body has carried you through every aspect of life. You can't hate yourself happy or criticize yourself thin. You have been criticizing yourself for years and it hasn't worked. *Be proud* of how your body has carried you through and move forward with gratitude.

BE CAREFUL WHAT YOU SAY, YOUR BODY IS LISTENING!

-Dr. Charryse

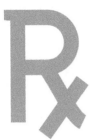

Prescription for: Growth

#lessismore

Date: Week 6

Patient: _____

Instructions:

Say NO without giving a long explanation or trying to sandwich your response to ensure you can still please others. If you need a little extra language, you can adjust. Simply say: "No, thankyou". LOL!

Refill script_____times

x - PRN NR

Sleep

I woke up feeling...   **Hrs:**

_____

_____   1 2 3 4 5 6 7 8+

_____

_____

_____

Review your day: **Water**

**What adjustments
to your schedule
would honor your
needs today?**

     16 16 16 16

     16 16 16 16

_____

_____

_____   Personal
development:

_____ _____

_____

**What do you want to
experience today?** _____

_____

_____ _____

_____

_____ _____

_____

Gratitude:

_____

_____

_____

_____

5 min of meditation,
stillness, or quiet

1 2   3   4   5

Be mindful of
your eating

_____

_____

_____

_____

Evaluate your day.
What went well
today?

_____

_____

_____

_____

Today my eating
motivation was to...

NOURISH

NUMB

Tomorrow I look
forward to...

_____

_____

_____

_____

☐   *used an accountability resource*

Daily Reflections

Scripture of the day:

Proverbs 28:1

Sleep

I woke up feeling...   **Hrs:**

_____

_____   1 2 3 4 5 6 7 8+

_____

_____

Review your day: **Water**

**What adjustments
to your schedule
would honor your
needs today?**

16 16 16 16

16 16 16 16

_____

_____

_____   Personal
                                        development:

**What do you want to
experience today?**

_____

_____

_____

_____

Gratitude:

_____
_____
_____
_____

5 min of meditation, stillness, or quiet

1 2   3 4 5

Be mindful of your eating

_____
_____
_____
_____

Evaluate your day. What went well today?

_____
_____
_____
_____

Today my eating motivation was to...

NOURISH

NUMB

Tomorrow I look forward to...

_____
_____
_____
_____

☐ *used an accountability resource*

Daily Reflections

_____

_____

_____

_____

_____

_____

_____

_____

_____

_____

_____

Scripture of the day:

Psalm 31:24

Sleep

I woke up feeling...   **Hrs:**

_____

_____   1 2 3 4 5 6 7 8+

_____

_____

Review your day: **Water**

**What adjustments
to your schedule**   16 16 16 16
**would honor your
needs today?**   16 16 16 16

_____

_____

_____   Personal
                                             development:
_____

                                     _____

What do you want to   _____
experience today?
                                     _____
_____
                                     _____
_____
                                     _____
_____
                                     _____
_____

_____

Gratitude:

_____

_____

_____

5 min of meditation, stillness, or quiet

1 2   3   4   5

Be mindful of your eating

_____

_____

_____

_____

Evaluate your day. What went well today?

_____

_____

_____

_____

Today my eating motivation was to...

NOURISH

NUMB

Tomorrow I look forward to...

_____

_____

_____

_____

☐   *used an accountability resource*

Daily Reflections

_____

_____

_____

_____

_____

_____

_____

_____

_____

_____

_____

Scripture of the day:

Psalm 112:7

Sleep

I woke up feeling...   **Hrs:**

_____

_____   1 2 3 4 5 6 7 8+

_____

_____

Review your day: **Water**

**What adjustments
to your schedule
would honor your
needs today?**   16 16 16 16

                                          16 16 16 16

_____

_____

_____   Personal
                                                         development:

_____

**What do you want to   _____
experience today?**
                                       _____

_____   _____

_____   _____

_____   _____

_____   _____

Gratitude:

_____

_____

_____

_____

5 min of meditation, stillness, or quiet

1 2   3 4 5

Be mindful of your eating

_____

_____

_____

Evaluate your day. What went well today?

_____

_____

_____

Today my eating motivation was to...

NOURISH

NUMB

Tomorrow I look forward to...

_____

_____

_____

_____

☐   *used an accountability resource*

Daily Reflections

Scripture of the day:

1 Chronicles 28:20

Sleep

I woke up feeling...

Hrs:

_____

_____

1 2 3 4 5 6 7 8+

_____

_____

Review your day:

Water

What adjustments to your schedule would honor your needs today?

16 16 16 16

16 16 16 16

_____

_____

_____

_____

Personal development:

What do you want to experience today?

_____

_____

_____

_____

_____

_____

_____

Gratitude:

_____

_____

_____

5 min of meditation,
stillness, or quiet

1 2   3   4   5

*Be mindful of
your eating*

_____

_____

_____

_____

**Evaluate your day.
What went well
today?**

_____

_____

_____

_____

**Today my eating
motivation was to...**

NOURISH

NUMB

Tomorrow I look
forward to...

_____

_____

_____

_____

☐   *used an accountability resource*

Daily Reflections

_____

_____

_____

_____

_____

_____

_____

_____

_____

Scripture of the day:

Psalm 27:12-14

Sleep

I woke up feeling...

Hrs:

_____
_____
_____
_____
_____

1 2 3 4 5 6 7 8+

Review your day:

Water

What adjustments
to your schedule
would honor your
needs today?

16 16 16 16

16 16 16 16

_____
_____
_____
_____

Personal
development:

_____

**What do you want to
experience today?**

_____
_____
_____
_____
_____
_____
_____
_____
_____

Gratitude:

_____

_____

_____

5 min of meditation,
stillness, or quiet

1 2   3 4 5

*Be mindful of
your eating*

_____

_____

_____

**Evaluate your day.
What went well
today?**

_____

_____

_____

**Today my eating
motivation was to...**

NOURISH

NUMB

Tomorrow I look
forward to...

_____

_____

_____

_____

☐   *used an accountability resource*

Daily Reflections

_____

_____

_____

_____

_____

_____

_____

_____

_____

_____

Scripture of the day:

Hebrews 10:25

Sleep

I woke up feeling...

Hrs:

_____

_____

1 2 3 4 5 6 7 8+

_____

_____

Review your day:

Water

What adjustments
to your schedule
would honor your
needs today?

16 16 16 16

16 16 16 16

_____

_____

_____

_____

Personal
development:

_____

What do you want to
experience today?

_____

_____

_____

_____

_____

_____

_____

_____

Gratitude:

_____

_____

_____

_____

5 min of meditation,
stillness, or quiet

1 2   3   4   5

Be mindful of
your eating

_____

_____

_____

_____

Evaluate your day.
What went well
today?

_____

_____

_____

_____

Today my eating
motivation was to...

NOURISH

NUMB

Tomorrow I look
forward to...

_____

_____

_____

_____

☐   *used an accountability resource*

Daily Reflections

Scripture of the day:

Joshua 1:9

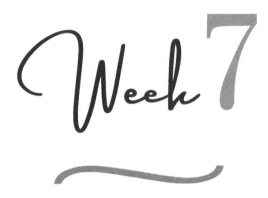

Doctor's *Note*

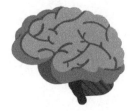

There are two kinds of guilt: the kind that drowns you until you're useless, and the kind that fires your soul to purpose.

WHICH ONE WILL YOU CHOOSE?

—Dr. Charryse

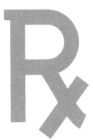

Prescription for: Growth

#socialbrain

___

Date: Week 7

Patient: _____

Instructions:

Spend time reconnecting with someone that you enjoy but don't get to see often. If possible, engage in this time face-to-face. This will allow you to practice co-regulation and experience the feeling of your body at ease.

Refill script_____times

x – PRN NR

Sleep

I woke up feeling...

Hrs:

_____

_____

1 2 3 4 5 6 7 8+

_____

_____

Review your day:

Water

What adjustments to your schedule would honor your needs today?

16 16 16 16

16 16 16 16

_____

_____

_____

_____

Personal development:

What do you want to experience today?

_____

_____

_____

_____

_____

_____

_____

_____

_____

Gratitude:

_____

_____

_____

5 min of meditation,
stillness, or quiet

1 2   3   4   5

_Be mindful of
your eating_

_____

_____

_____

_____

**Evaluate your day.
What went well
today?**

_____

_____

_____

_____

**Today my eating
motivation was to...**

NOURISH

NUMB

Tomorrow I look
forward to...

_____

_____

_____

_____

☐   _used an accountability resource_

Daily Reflections

Scripture of the day:

Joshua 10:25

Sleep

I woke up feeling...   **Hrs:**

_____
_____   1 2 3 4 5 6 7 8+
_____
_____

Review your day: **Water**

**What adjustments
to your schedule
would honor your
needs today?**   16 16 16 16

                        16 16 16 16

_____
_____
_____
_____
                                    Personal
                                    development:

**What do you want to
experience today?**
_____
_____
_____
_____
_____
_____
_____
_____

Gratitude:

_____

_____

_____

_____

5 min of meditation, stillness, or quiet

1 2   3   4   5

Be mindful of your eating

_____

_____

_____

_____

Evaluate your day. What went well today?

_____

_____

_____

Today my eating motivation was to...

NOURISH

NUMB

Tomorrow I look forward to...

_____

_____

_____

_____

☐   *used an accountability resource*

Daily Reflections

_____

_____

_____

_____

_____

_____

_____

_____

_____

_____

Scripture of the day:

2 Corinthians 5:8

Sleep

I woke up feeling...

Hrs:

_____

_____

1 2 3 4 5 6 7 8+

_____

_____

Review your day:

Water

What adjustments to your schedule would honor your needs today?

16 16 16 16

16 16 16 16

_____

_____

_____

Personal development:

_____

What do you want to experience today?

_____

_____

_____

_____

_____

_____

_____

_____

_____

Gratitude:

_____

_____

_____

5 min of meditation,
stillness, or quiet

1 2   3 4 5

*Be mindful of
your eating*

_____

_____

_____

_____

**Evaluate your day.
What went well
today?**

_____

_____

_____

_____

**Today my eating
motivation was to...**

NOURISH

NUMB

Tomorrow I look
forward to...

_____

_____

_____

_____

☐   *used an accountability resource*

Daily Reflections

_____

_____

_____

_____

_____

_____

_____

_____

_____

_____

_____

Scripture of the day:

Deuteronomy 31:23

Sleep

I woke up feeling...

Hrs:

_____
_____

1 2 3 4 5 6 7 8+

_____
_____

Review your day:

Water

What adjustments
to your schedule
would honor your
needs today?

16 16 16 16

16 16 16 16

_____
_____
_____
_____

Personal
development:

_____

**What do you want to
experience today?**

_____
_____
_____
_____
_____
_____

Gratitude:

_____

_____

_____

_____

5 min of meditation, stillness, or quiet

1 2 3 4 5

Be mindful of your eating

_____

_____

_____

_____

Evaluate your day. What went well today?

_____

_____

_____

_____

Today my eating motivation was to...

NOURISH

NUMB

Tomorrow I look forward to...

_____

_____

_____

_____

☐   *used an accountability resource*

Daily Reflections

_____

_____

_____

_____

_____

_____

_____

_____

_____

_____

Scripture of the day:

Matthew 17:20

Sleep

I woke up feeling...

Hrs:

_____

_____

1 2 3 4 5 6 7 8+

_____

_____

_____

Review your day:

Water

**What adjustments
to your schedule
would honor your
needs today?**

16 16 16 16

16 16 16 16

_____

_____

_____

Personal
development:

_____

**What do you want to
experience today?**

_____

_____

_____

_____

_____

_____

_____

_____

Gratitude:

_____

_____

_____

_____

5 min of meditation,
stillness, or quiet

1　2　3　4　5

_Be mindful of
your eating_

_____

_____

_____

_____

**Evaluate your day.
What went well
today?**

_____

_____

_____

_____

**Today my eating
motivation was to...**

NOURISH

NUMB

Tomorrow I look
forward to...

_____

_____

_____

_____

☐　　_used an accountability resource_

Daily Reflections

Scripture of the day:

Hebrews 13:5-6

Sleep

I woke up feeling...

Hrs:

_____

_____

1 2 3 4 5 6 7 8+

_____

_____

Review your day:

Water

What adjustments
to your schedule
would honor your
needs today?

16 16 16 16

16 16 16 16

_____

_____

Personal
development:

_____

**What do you want to
experience today?**

_____

_____

_____

_____

_____

_____

_____

_____

Gratitude:

_____

_____

_____

_____

5 min of meditation, stillness, or quiet

1　2　3　4　5

Be mindful of your eating

_____

_____

_____

_____

Evaluate your day. What went well today?

_____

_____

_____

_____

Today my eating motivation was to...

NOURISH

NUMB

Tomorrow I look forward to...

_____

_____

_____

_____

☐　　_used an accountability resource_

Daily Reflections

_____

_____

_____

_____

_____

_____

_____

_____

_____

_____

_____

_____

Scripture of the day:

Joshua 2:11

Sleep

I woke up feeling...

Hrs:

_____

_____   1 2 3 4 5 6 7 8+

_____

_____

Review your day:

Water

What adjustments to your schedule would honor your needs today?

16 16 16 16

16 16 16 16

_____

_____

_____

Personal

_____   development:

_____

What do you want to experience today?

_____

_____

_____

_____

_____

_____

_____

_____

_____

_____

Gratitude:

_____

_____

_____

_____

5 min of meditation,
stillness, or quiet

1 2   3   4   5

*Be mindful of
your eating*

_____

_____

_____

_____

**Evaluate your day.
What went well
today?**

_____

_____

_____

_____

**Today my eating
motivation was to...**

NOURISH

NUMB

Tomorrow I look
forward to...

_____

_____

_____

_____

☐   *used an accountability resource*

Daily Reflections

_____

_____

_____

_____

_____

_____

_____

_____

_____

_____

Scripture of the day:

Isaiah 43:2

Week 8

Doctor's Note

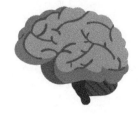

Don't fear what you're becoming! Even through the twists and turns, see yourself working through every challenge. You're either building, repairing, or fortifying the foundation of your health. Each season requires vision and trust in your efforts.

KEEP WORKING!!

—Dr. Charryse

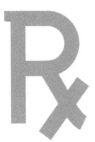

Prescription for: Growth

#findyourflow

Date: Week 8

Patient: _____

Instructions:

Plan a day date *by yourself*. Whether it's a few hours or most of the day, flow through the day and decide how *you* want to spend your time. The goal is to relax, do things you enjoy, and practice making choices that honor your needs.

Refill Script_____**times**

x – PRN NR

Sleep

I woke up feeling...   **Hrs:**

_____
_____   1 2 3 4 5 6 7 8+
_____
_____
_____

Review your day: **Water**

**What adjustments
to your schedule
would honor your
needs today?**   16 16 16 16

                                16 16 16 16

_____
_____
_____
_____
                                **Personal
                                development:**

**What do you want to   _____
experience today?**   _____

_____   _____
_____   _____
_____   _____
_____   _____

Gratitude:

_____

_____

_____

5 min of meditation,
stillness, or quiet

1 2   3 4 5

*Be mindful of
your eating*

_____

_____

_____

_____

**Evaluate your day.
What went well
today?**

_____

_____

_____

_____

**Today my eating
motivation was to...**

NOURISH

NUMB

Tomorrow I look
forward to...

_____

_____

_____

_____

☐   *used an accountability resource*

Daily Reflections

_____

_____

_____

_____

_____

_____

_____

_____

_____

_____

Scripture of the day:

Psalm 107:1

Sleep

I woke up feeling...   **Hrs:**

_____

_____   1 2 3 4 5 6 7 8+

_____

_____

Review your day: **Water**

What adjustments   16 16 16 16
to your schedule
would honor your   16 16 16 16
needs today?

_____

_____

_____   Personal
                                              development:
_____

                                       _____
What do you want to
experience today?   _____

_____   _____

_____   _____

_____   _____

_____   _____

Gratitude:

_____

_____

_____

5 min of meditation, stillness, or quiet

1 2   3 4 5

Be mindful of your eating

_____

_____

_____

Evaluate your day. What went well today?

_____

_____

_____

Today my eating motivation was to...

NOURISH

NUMB

Tomorrow I look forward to...

_____

_____

_____

_____

☐　　_used an accountability resource_

Daily Reflections

_____

_____

_____

_____

_____

_____

_____

_____

_____

_____

Scripture of the day:

1 Peter 5:7

Sleep

I woke up feeling...　　　　　　**Hrs:**

_____

_____　　1 2 3 4 5 6 7 8+

_____

_____

Review your day:　　　　　**Water**

**What adjustments
to your schedule
would honor your
needs today?**　　　16 16 16 16

　　　　　　　　　　16 16 16 16

_____

_____

_____　　　　　　**Personal
development:**

_____

**What do you want to
experience today?**
_____

_____

_____

_____

_____

_____

_____

_____

Gratitude:

_____

_____

_____

_____

5 min of meditation,
stillness, or quiet

1 2   3   4   5

_Be mindful of
your eating_

_____

_____

_____

_____

**Evaluate your day.
What went well
today?**

_____

_____

_____

_____

**Today my eating
motivation was to...**

NOURISH

NUMB

Tomorrow I look
forward to...

_____

_____

_____

_____

☐   _used an accountability resource_

Daily Reflections

Scripture of the day:

Proverbs 18:10

Sleep

I woke up feeling...

Hrs:

_____
_____
_____
_____
_____

1 2 3 4 5 6 7 8+

Review your day:

Water

What adjustments to your schedule would honor your needs today?

16 16 16 16

16 16 16 16

_____
_____
_____
_____

Personal
development:

_____

What do you want to experience today?

_____
_____
_____
_____
_____
_____
_____

Gratitude:

_____

_____

_____

5 min of meditation, stillness, or quiet

1 2 3 4 5

Be mindful of your eating

_____

_____

_____

_____

Evaluate your day. What went well today?

_____

_____

_____

Today my eating motivation was to...

NOURISH

NUMB

Tomorrow I look forward to...

_____

_____

_____

_____

☐   *used an accountability resource*

Daily Reflections

_____

_____

_____

_____

_____

_____

_____

_____

_____

_____

_____

Scripture of the day:

Psalm 27:4

Sleep

I woke up feeling...

Hrs:

_____

_____

1 2 3 4 5 6 7 8+

_____

_____

_____

Review your day:

Water

What adjustments to your schedule would honor your needs today?

16 16 16 16

16 16 16 16

_____

_____

_____

Personal development:

_____

What do you want to experience today?

_____

_____

_____

_____

_____

_____

_____

_____

_____

Gratitude:

_____

_____

_____

5 min of meditation,
stillness, or quiet

1 2   3   4   5

_Be mindful of
your eating_

_____

_____

_____

_____

**Evaluate your day.
What went well
today?**

_____

_____

_____

_____

**Today my eating
motivation was to...**

NOURISH

NUMB

Tomorrow I look
forward to...

_____

_____

_____

_____

☐   _used an accountability resource_

Daily Reflections

_____

_____

_____

_____

_____

_____

_____

_____

_____

_____

Scripture of the day:

Isaiah 40:31

Sleep

I woke up feeling...   **Hrs:**

_____

_____   1 2 3 4 5 6 7 8+

_____

_____

Review your day: **Water**

**What adjustments
to your schedule
would honor your
needs today?**

16 16 16 16

16 16 16 16

_____

_____

_____   Personal
                                           development:

_____

**What do you want to
experience today?**

_____

_____

_____

_____

_____

Gratitude:

_____

_____

_____

5 min of meditation, stillness, or quiet

1 2   3 4 5

Be mindful of your eating

Evaluate your day. What went well today?

_____

_____

_____

_____

Today my eating motivation was to...

NOURISH

NUMB

Tomorrow I look forward to...

_____

_____

_____

☐ _used an accountability resource_

Daily Reflections

_____

_____

_____

_____

_____

_____

_____

_____

_____

_____

_____

Scripture of the day:

Romans 15:4

Sleep

I woke up feeling...

Hrs:

1 2 3 4 5 6 7 8+

_____

_____

_____

_____

_____

Review your day:

Water

What adjustments
to your schedule
would honor your
needs today?

16 16 16 16

16 16 16 16

_____

_____

_____

_____

Personal
development:

_____

**What do you want to
experience today?**

_____

_____

_____

_____

_____

_____

_____

_____

_____

Gratitude:

_____

_____

_____

5 min of meditation,
stillness, or quiet

1 2   3   4   5

*Be mindful of
your eating*

_____

_____

_____

_____

**Evaluate your day.
What went well
today?**

_____

_____

_____

_____

**Today my eating
motivation was to...**

NOURISH

NUMB

*Tomorrow I look
forward to...*

_____

_____

_____

_____

☐   *used an accountability resource*

Daily Reflections

_____

_____

_____

_____

_____

_____

_____

_____

_____

_____

Scripture of the day:

Mark 10:27

Doctor's Note

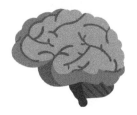

Change requires focus. This can mean distancing yourself from anyone or anything that drains your focus. You are NOT a victim. Don't sit back and let people speak doubt into your journey.

REFUSE TO BE DEFEATED!

-Dr. Charryse